Free To Dance & Think Again

64+ YEARS TYPE I DIABETES &
NO NEUROPATHY OR RETINOPATHY
FREE FROM PARKINSON'S DISEASE & MIRAPEX:
METHODOLOGY & THEORY

by
William Kelly Dagenhart, PhD

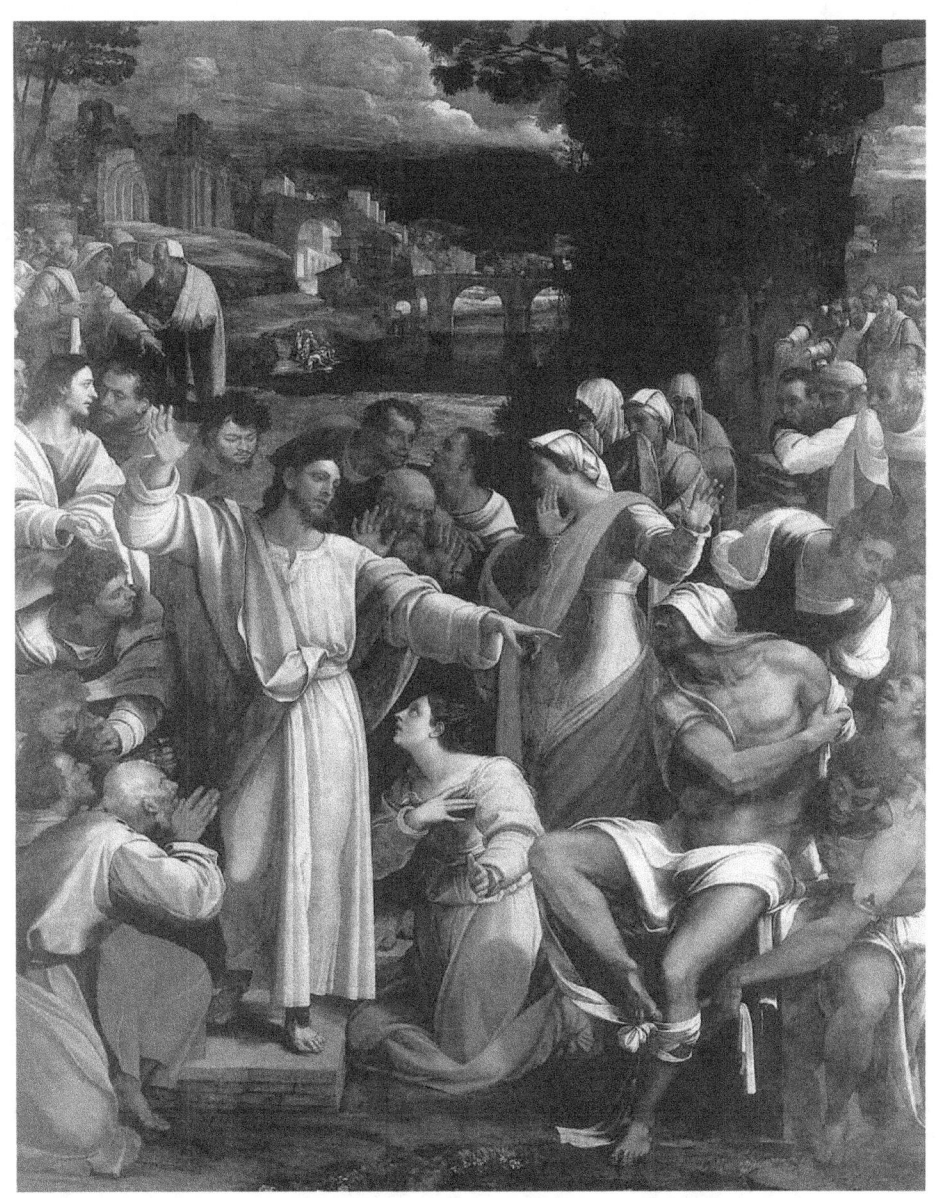

**Raising of Lazarus was painted
by Sebastiano del Piombo I (1485?-1547) in 1517-1519**

ISBN: 1499738579
ISBN 13: 9781499738575

FOREWORD

I HAVE BEEN INSPIRED SINCE CHILDHOOD BY THE WORDS FROM THE HOLY SCRIPTURES THAT YOUR BODY IS THE TEMPLE OF GOD AND HAVE CONTINUED TO ACT ON THIS INSPIRATION.[1]

---

[1] **1 Corinthians 6:19-20, Your Body, His Temple**

"Do you not know that your body is a temple of the Holy Spirit, who is in you, whom you have received from God? You are not your own; you were bought at a price. Therefore honor God with your body," (1 Cor. 6:19-20), from ROMANS COMMENTARY, the Moody Bible Commentary.

Only through Jesus Christ and many others was this Miracle possible!

TABLE OF CONTENTS

Only through Jesus Christ and many others was this Miracle possible!

INSPIRATION

A DREAM FROM GOD

A Hugely Successful Lifelong Health Experiment and NEW HEALTH THEORIES & PLANS by a devoted Oak Ridge First United Methodist Church Christian[2] – A Physicist retired from The Oak Ridge National Laboratory

$$\infty + \Omega$$

A RECENT PROGRESSING MIRACLE OF GOD – GETTING FREE FROM PARKINSON'S DISEASE & THE TERRIBLE MEDICATION PRESCRIBED FOR ME TO COMBAT IT – MIRAPEX.

This first book is to tell my story of getting rid of much of the debilitating part of Parkinson's and one of its medicines Mirapex, an event which has been a huge improvement for me and my family. I claim that this bad Mirapex experience may be true for many more. Statistically, I just know of too many very bad experiences myself, in my friends and acquaintances. I am seeking to get support to test this assertion on a group of 100 Parkinson's patients in order to get good statistics. I estimate that more than 80% of Parkinson's patients, who are having my kind of troubles, will achieve my results upon applying my methods. The method of aerobic[3] exercise instead of the debilitating Mirapex medicine is simple and can be used all around the world for even the poorest peoples. All exercises must be used to get or keep flexibility and strength in

---

[2] *The huge influence of Faith in God on Health is recounted in a large number of books, magazines, newspaper articles, and health publications. One mate dies and the other closely follows within a week or so. The hospital of the future has many instances of combating loneliness. In my current terrible health journey due to Parkinson's and its medication MIRAPEX, I have been supported by God in this journey, which has overwhelmed many. My family was very supportive, but did not know themselves the outcome. The Great Healer, JESUS CHRIST, held me and my family up. Then our workers, our extended family living away, and our other family members came in with tremendous support. WE SIMPLY MUST PROVIDE THIS SUPPORT FOR FAMILIES THAT HAVE NOT BEEN BROUGHT TO GOD IN JESUS CHRIST AND/OR HAVE NO FAMILY SUPPORT. Our family is available to help anybody tackling these tasks of faith and life. This includes our opinions on the medical journey I am having.*

Only through Jesus Christ and many others was this Miracle possible!

addition to the aerobic exercises and should be used throughout life, and can be started now for everybody without any exceptions. This better health method is like forgiveness from our Lord; it can always be accepted now. The exercise level and effort required to get aerobic is different for different people and varies as your physical condition improves. The methods to get aerobic and physically fit vary as you get more physically fit and with your economic conditions. This Taking Care of God's Temple must be a lifelong process. I also think that this method should be rapidly tested for its applicability to such other diseases as Alzheimer's, dementia, fibromyalgia, and others. My theory for cause and treatment says that the methods I use are applicable to all these neurological diseases. At the very least, more exercise will make The United States' citizens healthier and bring about weight loss. Weight is now increasing among so many. Our families that we came from and our present nuclear family has always been concerned about nutrition and what it is that we eat. Data continues to be gathered about what to eat and it is now very experimentally plain that what we eat does matter. I just saw a program on National Public Television[4] that confirms our family's lifelong thoughts on nutrition. There are huge increases in probabilities of surviving or never having certain diseases by using proper nutrition.

//

FROM THE NEW TESTAMENT[5]

The Story of Jesus Christ Raising Lazarus from the Dead

Now a certain man was ill, Lazarus of Bethany, the village of Mary and her sister Martha. It was Mary who anointed the Lord with ointment and who wiped his feet with her hair, whose brother Lazarus was ill. So the sisters sent to him, saying, "Lord, he whom you love is ill." But when Jesus heard it he said, "This illness is not unto death, it is for the glory of God, so that the Son of God may be glorified by means of it." Now Jesus loved Martha and her sister and Lazarus. So when he heard that he was ill, he stayed two days longer in the place where he was. Then after this he said to the disciples, "Let us go into Judea again." The disciples said to him, "Rabbi, the Jews were but now seeking to stone you, and are you going there again?" Jesus answered, "Are

---

[4] *I refer you to National Public Television and a huge number of other sources of information on the latest research and data on nutrition.*

[5] *From "THE NEW OXFORD ANNOTATED BIBLE WITH THE APOCRYPHA", expanded edition, an ecumenical study Bible – REVISED STANDARD VERSION. ISBN 0-19-528348-1.*

there not twelve hours in the day? If anyone walks in the day, he does not stumble, because he sees the light of this world. But if anyone walks in the night, he stumbles, because the light is not in him." Thus he spoke, and then he said to them, "Our friend Lazarus has fallen asleep, but I go to wake him out of sleep." The disciples said to him, "Lord, if he has fallen asleep, he will recover."

Now Jesus had spoken of his death, but they thought that he meant taking rest in sleep. Then Jesus told them plainly, "Lazarus is dead, and for your sake I am glad that I was not there, so that you may believe. But let us go to him." Thomas, called the Twin, said to his fellow disciples, "Let us also go, that we may die with him." Now when Jesus came, he found that Lazarus had already been in the tomb four days. Bethany was near Jerusalem, about two miles off, and many of the Jews had come to Martha and Mary to console them concerning their brother. When Martha heard that Jesus was coming, she went and met him, while Mary set in the house. Martha said to Jesus, "Lord, if you had been here, my brother would not have died. And even now I know that whatever you ask from God, God will give you." Jesus said to her, "Your brother will rise again." Martha said to him, "I know that he will rise again in the resurrection at the last day."

Jesus said to her, "I am the resurrection and the Life, he who believes in me, though he die, yet shall he live and whoever lives and believes in me shall never die. Do you believe this?" She said to him, "Yes, Lord I believe that you are the Christ, the Son of God, he who is coming into the world." When she had said this, she went and called her sister Mary, saying quietly, "The teacher is here and is calling for you." And when she heard it, she rose quickly and went to him. Now Jesus had not yet come to the village, but was still in the place where Martha had met him. When the Jews, who were with her in the house, consoling her, saw Mary rise quickly and go out, they followed her, supposing that she was going to the tomb to weep there. Then Mary, when she came to where Jesus was and saw him, fell at his feet, saying to him, "Lord, if you had been here, my brother would not have died." When Jesus saw her weeping, and the Jews who came with her also weeping, he was deeply moved in spirit and troubled, and he said, "Where have you laid him?" They said to him, "Lord, come and see."

Jesus wept. So the Jews said. "See how he loved him!" But some of them said. "Could not he who opened the eyes of the blind man have kept this man from dying?" Then Jesus, deeply moved again, came to the tomb, it was a cave, and a stone lay upon it. Jesus said, "Take away the stone." Martha, the sister of the dead man, said to him, "Lord, by this time there will be an odor, for he has been dead four days. Jesus said to her, "Did I not tell you that if you would believe you would see the glory of God?" So they took away the stone. And Jesus lifted up his eyes and said, "Father, I thank thee that thou hast heard me. I knew that thou hearest me always, but I have said this on the account of the people standing by, that they may believe that thou didst send me." When he had said this, he cried with a loud voice, "Lazarus, come out." The dead man came out, his hands and feet bound with bandages, and his face wrapped with a cloth. Jesus said to them "Unbind him and let him go."   John 11:1-44

What do the Scriptures say we can do?

The Way, the Truth, and the Life
..."*Believe Me that I am in the Father and the Father is in Me; otherwise believe because of the works themselves. "Truly, truly, I say to you, he who believes in Me, the works that I do, he will do also; and greater works than these he will do; because I go to the Father." Whatever you ask in My name, that will I do, so that the Father may be glorified in the Son...."* John 14:11-13

///

I know of many family and personal friends who were in conditions with Parkinson's disease like mine and they died. I was at pain level 10 in the fall of 2012 and at that time thought that I was dead. Not very many survive this condition.

///

SUPPORT THAT I HAVE HAD AND STILL HAVE IN THESE HEALTH STRUGGLES

My progress was made possible by many things, including -

- Enduring faith in God and Jesus Christ Son of God, since earliest childhood taught to me to by my loving parents.
- My devoted and loving wife of 57 years, Sally, who has worshiped with me and led our family to worship.
- DayBreak Personal Services -- headed by my loving daughter, Pamela L. Dagenhart, and her entire staff – especially office staff members Monica Carlisle and Paige Harmon.
- The Internet – a source of all published medical experiments and literature that led me to the methods used now and supports many of the methods, which I have used all my life, starting before 1949, long before the internet.
- Medical staff of diverse locations, who said my methods were acceptable, but maybe were not as quite optimistic as I was -- especially doctors Elaine Bunick and James Burns.
- Retired Internal Medicine Doctor Verne Gilbert – My hero, who himself is beset by health problems, but who came to my next door home office to talk and tell me that I was free from Parkinson's disease.
- Also to be noted is the fact that Doctor Verne Gilbert came immediately in his coat-covered pajamas to respond to my severe heart attack at 7 AM on April 6, 1993 at my home in Oak Ridge, TN. The response to the emergency 911 call placed by my wife, and response by police, fire truck, and ambulance personnel

Only through Jesus Christ and many others was this Miracle possible!

was so fast, that I was being loaded into the ambulance within about 5 minutes from the emergency call. The heart attack happened as I was shaving, in preparation for work at The Oak Ridge National Laboratory. The heart attack felt like someone had drop-kicked me in the chest. Doctor Gilbert helped our wonderful ambulance crew do a pre-departure evaluation and I was quickly transported.

- The thankfulness of a quick heart attack response also goes gratefully and lovingly to all at Oak Ridge Methodist Hospital staff, now a part of Covenant Health, a multi-hospital local organization. Emergency Room Doctor, Jim Henry, got the ER quickly in operation and then my heart Doctor, Jim Michel, took over. Jim took over and did an expansion of my left anterior descending heart artery that was almost closed up! Stents were only a few months away to be in regular use, but without one I have done well. My father had his first heart attack at 46 and his fatal one at age 54. Thank God to all the medical personnel who made the new heart treatment advances possible.

- Recently seen on the Public Television show on Channel 2 with 'Doctor Bob' Overholt was a feature with Dr. Wolfe J. Frederick, MD of Rheumatology Associates of Knoxville, TN. Doctor Frederick is using aerobic exercise and other exercises to battle his fibromyalgia. My daughter, Pamela Dagenhart owner of DayBreak Personal Services of Oak Ridge, TN is planning to use some of these techniques, which I and Doctor Frederick use, to get rid of her fibromyalgia symptoms. We are planning to work with local doctors to get rid of her fibromyalgia and then plan to expand the demonstration to make that a main treatment for fibromyalgia.

- This is some of the recent research literature and use, which supports my lifelong methods.

//

Acknowledgements

Dealing with these problems with Parkinson's disease, has put huge stresses on my family. In many other family cases, the use of Mirapex has caused similar stresses to other families even to the point of break ups. This statement is supported by the large class action law suits won in the state of California against the Mirapex manufacturer, Boehringer Ingelheim Pharmaceuticals, Inc. We know of some very bad Mirapex experiences that patients have had in Tennessee also, but do not have an accurate count yet.

To put the deaths of Parkinson's patients in some perspective I have gathered the following data from United States Government Health agencies. In 2009, a total of 2,437,163 deaths were reported in the United States. From The Parkinson's Action Network we get CDC reported data on Parkinson's for 2010, "As our population ages, legislation such as the National Neurological Diseases Surveillance System Act – coupled with strong federal funding overall for research and supportive policies for people and families living with Parkinson's disease – becomes ever more important. Between 500,000 and 1.5 million Americans live with Parkinson's, a disease for which there is no cure or treatment to stop the progression." The United States total population in 2010 by census was 308,745,538.

There are about 60,000 deaths of patients with Parkinson's each year in the United States.

I want to again especially express my profound thank you to my family, my wife Sally R. Dagenhart, and my daughter Pamela L. Dagenhart. I also want to express thanks to Pamela's office staff in our home/business office of DayBreak Personal Services, Monica Carlisle and Paige Harmon. All of them were involved in taking me to the many doctor's appointments, to physical therapy, and for the many laboratory tests.

All were patient with my greatly diminished performance in doing my Chief Financial Officer duties for DayBreak Personal Services and in cleaning up my messes.

Thanks also go to my former Oak Ridge National Laboratory Fusion Energy Boss, Dr. William Stirling and his wife Bobbie, who many times listened and took me to their Saturday Night Contemporary Worship Services. Thanks also go to the Oak Ridge First United Methodist Church home visitation minister Rev. Jenny Caughman, and the Stephen Ministry team of our Church.

Thanks also go out to Brian Matheney, who owns and operates a yard and landscaping business in Oak Ridge. He has provided the bulk of my transportation to my Oak Ridge First United Methodist Church Services and dinners. He also had been invaluable in keeping Remove Intoxicated Drivers of Oak Ridge/Anderson County operating by being on the Board of Directors, providing his pickup and large panel truck when needed for over 6 years.

Author – Dr. William Kelly Dagenhart and my wife of 57 years, Sally R. Dagenhart on upper left. To the upper right, our daughter Pamela L. Dagenhart, right, who lives with us and runs her DayBreak Personal Services home caregiving business from our office. Shown also with Pam from right to left are Sally, our lovely daughter-law Natasha Dagenhart, and her son Sergei Dubovov.

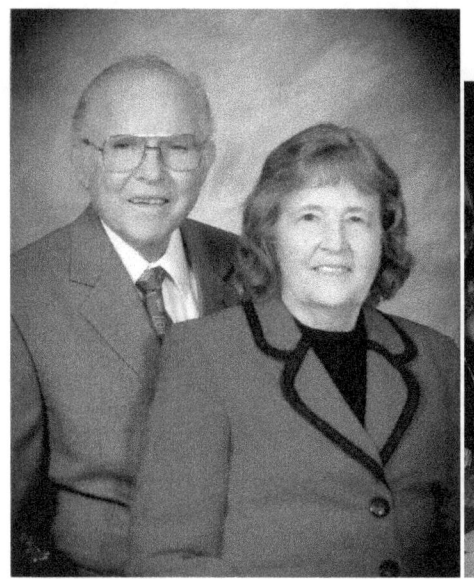
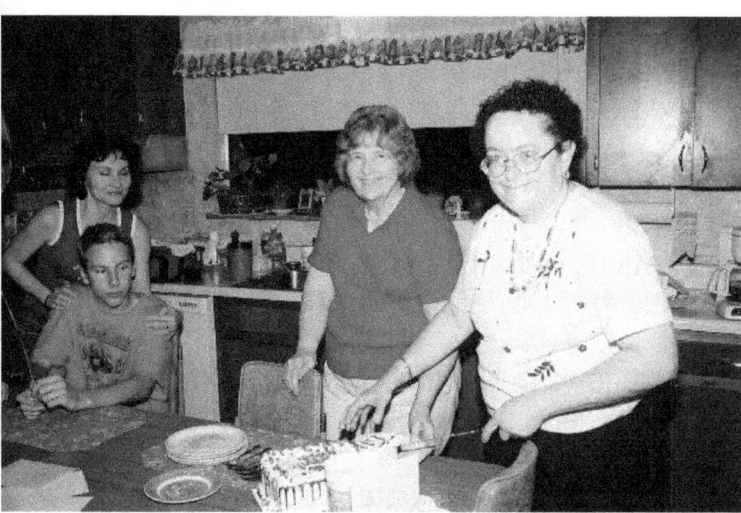

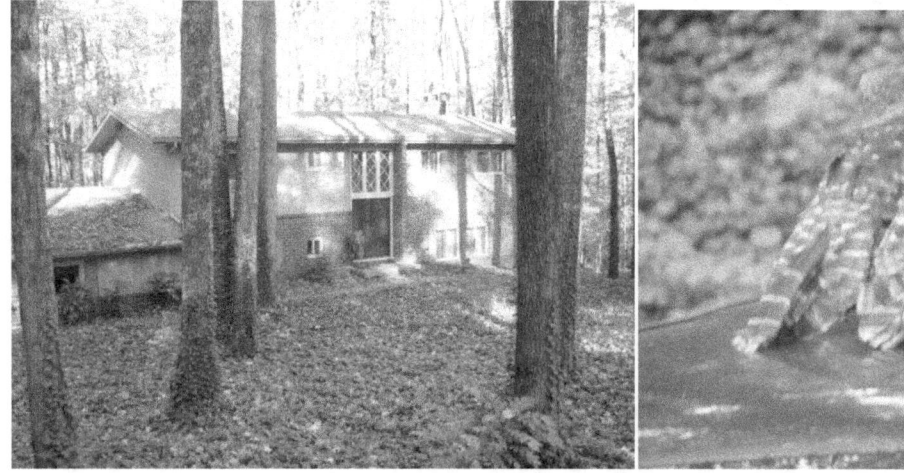
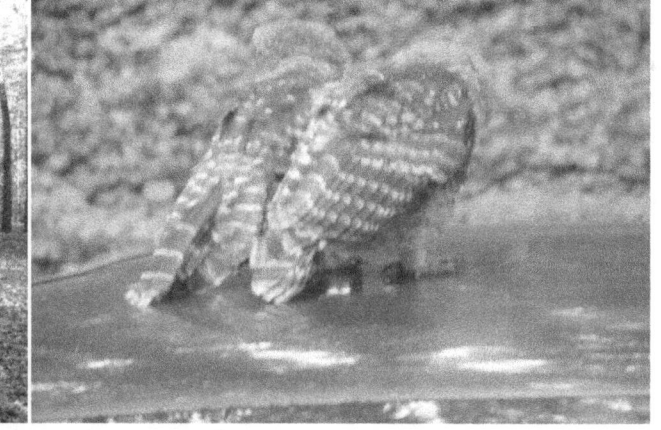

Our home that provides the support, help, and solitude needed to make this Medical Miracle of God possible with two locals, a family of owls, keeping watch from their vantage point atop our car.

SUMMARY OF THE TASK OF DEFEATING PARKINSON'S DISEASE

FROM THE PARKINSON'S DISEASE FOUNDATION

Causes

What Causes Parkinson's?

To date, despite decades of intensive study, the causes of Parkinson's Disease(PD) remain unknown. Many experts think that the disease is caused by a combination of genetic and environmental factors, which may vary from person to person.

In some people, genetic factors may play a role; in others, illness, an environmental toxin or other event may contribute to PD. Scientists have identified aging as an important risk factor; there is a two to four percent risk for PD among people over age 60, compared with one to two percent in the general population.

The chemical or genetic trigger that starts the cell death process in dopamine neurons is the subject of intense scientific study. Many believe that by understanding the sequence of events that leads to the loss of dopamine cells, scientists will be able to develop treatments to stop or reverse the disease.

Statistics on Parkinson's

Who Has Parkinson's?

- As many as one million Americans live with PD, which is more than the combined number of people diagnosed with multiple sclerosis, muscular dystrophy and Lou Gehrig's disease.
- Approximately 60,000 Americans are diagnosed with PD each year, and this number does not reflect the thousands of cases that go undetected.
- An estimated seven to ten million people worldwide are living with PD.
- Incidence of PD increases with age, but an estimated four percent of people with PD are diagnosed before the age of 50.
- Men are one and a half times more likely to have PD than women.

Only through Jesus Christ and many others was this Miracle possible!

What Does Parkinson's Cost?

- The combined direct and indirect cost of Parkinson's, including treatment, Social Security payments and lost income from inability to work, is estimated to be nearly $25 billion per year in the United States alone.
- Medication costs for an individual person with PD average $2,500 a year and therapeutic surgery can cost up to $100,000 dollars per patient.

Medications & Treatments

- There are many medications available to treat the symptoms of Parkinson's, although none yet that actually reverse the effects of the disease.

- It is common for people with PD to take a variety of these medications – all at different doses and at different times of day - in order to manage the symptoms of the disease.

- While keeping track of medications can be a challenging task, understanding your medications and sticking to a schedule will provide the greatest benefit from the drugs and avoid unpleasant "off" periods due to missed doses.

///

FROM THE NATIONAL INSTITUTE OF NEUROLOGICAL DISORDERS AND STROKES (NINDS)

What is Parkinson's Disease?

Historical View

Parkinson's disease is a progressive neurological disorder that results from degeneration of neurons in a region of the brain that controls movement. This degeneration creates a shortage of the brain signaling chemical (neurotransmitter) known as dopamine, causing the movement impairments that characterize the disease. Parkinson's disease was first formally described in "An Essay on the Shaking Palsy," published in 1817 by a London physician named James Parkinson, but it has probably existed for many thousands of years. Its symptoms and potential therapies were mentioned in the Ayurveda, the system of medicine practiced in India as early as 5000 BC, and in the first Chinese medical text, Nei Jing, which appeared 2500 years ago.

Difference Between Nerve and Neuron

• *Categorized under Science | Difference Between Nerve and Neuron*

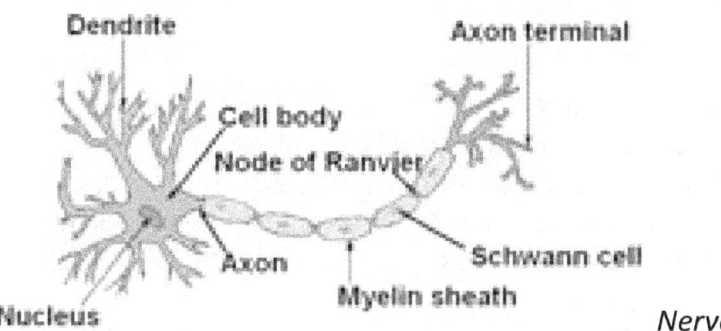

Nerve vs. Neuron

Although nerve and neuron may sound similar to most people, they are, in fact, two different components of the body. However, they are closely related, as nerves are actually projections of neurons.

There are three main types of nerves: Afferent nerves, efferent nerves, and mixed nerves. Afferent nerves transmit signals from sensory neurons to the central nervous system; efferent nerves transmit signals from the central nervous system to the muscles and glands, and mixed nerves are responsible for receiving sensory information, and for sending information to the muscles. Nerves are also classified as spinal nerves and cranial nerves. The spinal nerves connect the spinal column to the spinal cord, and transmit signals to most of the body, while cranial nerves are found in the brainstem, and they are responsible for the signals to the brain.

The nerve is composed of different types of axons, and it is through these axons that the electrochemical nerve impulses (mentioned above) are transmitted. Nerves are found in the peripheral nervous system. Each nerve is covered by three layers, starting with the inner endoneurium, which covers the nerve fibres; the middle layer called the perineurium, and the outer layer over the perineurium, called the epineurium. There are even blood vessels found within a nerve.

On the other hand, neurons are found in the brain, spinal cord and peripheral nerves. Neurons are also named as neurone, or as nerve cells. There are two types of neurons - the sensory neurons and the motor neurons. Sensory neurons send signals to the brain and the spinal cord, while the motor neurons receive signals from the brain and spinal cord. Therefore, information is transmitted through neurons by electrochemical signaling.

Neurons consist of various parts including the soma, nucleus, extensions called the dendrite tree, and the many axons. The soma is the central part of the neuron, and the nucleus is found within the soma. Dendrites form extensions from the neuron, and axons are the extensions from the soma. Axons are fine structures, and they vary in number from hundreds to thousands. The axon terminals have synapses, and the axon hillock is where the axon emerges from the soma.

Various diseases can occur when there is damage sustained to the nerves or the neurons. Nerve damage may lead to diseases such as carpal tunnel syndrome, immunological diseases like Guillain-Barre syndrome, and neuritis, which is when the nerves become infected. Diabetes could also cause nerve damage, and neuropathy refers to the damage of the blood vessels covering the nerves. Symptoms of the above-mentioned diseases include paralysis, pain, numbness and weakness of the nerves. In some cases, there is even referred pain in a different part of the body due to the damage of certain nerves.

<u>Alzheimer's, Charcott Marie Tooth, Myasthenia Gravis, and Parkinson's diseases are all caused by damage to the neurons.</u> Symptoms of these diseases include short-term memory loss, loss of sensory perception, agnosia, apraxia, aphasia, akinesia, tremors, muscle rigidity, bradykinesia, and many others.

Summary:

1. A neuron is an individual cell, whereas, a group of neurons form a nerve.
2. There are two types of neurons: sensory and motor neurons; while there are three types of nerves: afferent, efferent and mixed nerves.
3. Nerves are found in the peripheral nervous system, while neurons are found in the brain, spinal cord and the peripheral nerves.
4. A neuron can also be called a neurone or a nerve cell.
5. Neurons conduct nerve impulses, while nerves transmit information to various parts of the body.

Read more: *Difference Between Nerve and Neuron | Difference Between | Nerve vs Neuron* http://www.differencebetween.net/science/difference-between-nerve-and-neuron/#ixzz325ovIFQr

Alzheimer's Disease from
The Alzheimer's Foundation of America

About Alzheimer's

Definition

Alzheimer's disease is a progressive, degenerative disorder that attacks the brain's nerve cells, or neurons, resulting in loss of memory, thinking and language skills, and behavioral changes.

- These neurons, which produce the brain chemical or neurotransmitter, acetylcholine, break connections with other nerve cells and ultimately die. For example, short-term memory fails when Alzheimer's disease first destroys nerve cells in the hippocampus, and language skills and judgment decline when neurons die in the cerebral cortex.

- Two types of abnormal lesions clog the brains of individuals with Alzheimer's disease: Beta-amyloid plaques—sticky clumps of protein fragments and cellular material that form outside and around neurons; and neurofibrillary tangles—insoluble twisted fibers composed largely of the protein tau that build up inside nerve cells. Although these structures are hallmarks of the disease, scientists are unclear whether they cause it or a byproduct of it.

- Alzheimer's disease is the most common cause of dementia, or loss of intellectual function, among people aged 65 and older.

- Alzheimer's disease is not a normal part of aging.

- Origin of the term Alzheimer's disease dates back to 1906 when Dr. Alois Alzheimer, a German physician, presented a case history before a medical meeting of a 51-year-old woman who suffered from a rare brain disorder. A brain autopsy identified the plaques and tangles that today characterize Alzheimer's disease.

Fibromyalgia Data
A Disease which afflicts my Daughter

Data from the Mayo Clinic

Definition

Fibromyalgia is a disorder characterized by widespread musculoskeletal pain accompanied by fatigue, sleep, memory and mood issues. Researchers believe that fibromyalgia amplifies painful sensations by affecting the way your brain processes pain signals.

Symptoms sometimes begin after a physical trauma, surgery, infection or significant psychological stress. In other cases, symptoms gradually accumulate over time with no single triggering event.

Women are much more likely to develop fibromyalgia than are men. Many people who have fibromyalgia also have tension headaches, temporomandibular joint (TMJ) disorders, irritable bowel syndrome, anxiety and depression.

While there is no cure for fibromyalgia, a variety of medications can help control symptoms. Exercise, relaxation and stress-reduction measures also may help.

Causes

Doctors don't know what causes fibromyalgia, but it most likely involves a variety of factors working together. These may include:

- **Genetics** - Because fibromyalgia tends to run in families, there may be certain genetic mutations that may make you more susceptible to developing the disorder.

- **Infections** - Some illnesses appear to trigger or aggravate fibromyalgia.

- **Physical or emotional trauma** - Post-traumatic stress disorder has been linked to fibromyalgia.

Why does it hurt?

Researchers believe repeated nerve stimulation causes the brains of people with fibromyalgia to change. This change involves an abnormal increase in levels of certain chemicals in the brain that signal pain (neurotransmitters). In addition, the brain's pain receptors seem to develop a memory of the pain and become more sensitive, meaning they can, what would be in a non-pain syndrome sufferer overreact, to pain signals.

Only through Jesus Christ and many others was this Miracle possible!

Addendum on Treatment for Fibromyalgia from a local doctor's method of treatment and experience

My wife Sally and I saw a television show with Doctor Bob Overholt on National Public Television in May 2014 and his interviewee was Doctor Wolfe Frederick, Rheumatologist. Doctor Frederick has Fibromyalgia and follows the treatment and methods that should be used all one's life to keep many of these types of body damages from happening. He exercises aerobically and keeps his body in shape. At present we are seeking to get my daughter into this type of program for her fibromyalgia. She has been on other means of treatment that are not very effective and are expensive.

My own program is feeble due to financial constraints and support by the medical system. It has ramped up considerably during May 2014 and I should have conclusive results on how far in getting into better physical shape is possible for me. I was always convinced that this was the way for me, but conditions just prevented me from keeping up that level of physical activity. Very few supported my theory in this need for vigorous physical activity.

///

DAGENHART ADDITION TO PARKINSON'S THEORY AND TREATMENT

A. I hypothesize that the fundamental problem in Parkinson's and other similar diseases is caused by shortage of oxygen to the nerve/neuron system that leads to their degeneration. I hypothesize that this is mainly caused by low blood supply, which in turn is mostly caused by blood artery/vein narrowing. This shortage of blood supply can be caused by a number of things including, narrowing of the blood supply system by deposits of blood lipids, genetic narrow channels, and others. From hydraulics the blood supply can be increased by exercise, which should include aerobic levels to get maximum blood flow. The muscle/nerve systems call for increased heart rates for the muscles and this increase blood supply also to the nervous system. Staying physically fit is the first step in eliminating much of these problems.

B. What to do to prevent and/or cure these types of problems?
   1. Nerve damage of this type is prevented or cured by increasing the oxygen supply to the nerves that have been damaged.
   2. Increasing the oxygen supply can be accomplished by increased exercise rates. To do this the exercise should be done at aerobic rates. This exercise should be started by getting an evaluation from your cardiologist to set the safe exercise rates and should be reviewed periodically at times specified by the cardiologist. As exercise is increased for those who have not been active, the safe rate will increase to some maximum rate set by your heart pump and your blood system.
   3. I do know of heart attack victims that were not active, that after their heart attacks have gradually worked up in physical fitness and ran 25-mile marathons.
   4. My champion was a fellow in San Francisco, who jogged 5 miles per day and always ended up at a top class big restaurant. He was 105 years of age as last I have heard from him and he knew everybody at this restaurant and at 105 was hired as the maitre d'. He had lots of money, but this was fun for him.
   5. My projection is that if exercise is done lifelong, then the time at which you get into most health problems is moved out to greatly increased age and for many never. Death always comes, but on average your wellness will be good until very near death.
   6. In addition, Johns Hopkins Hospital has numerous publications showing that your basic brain functioning is greatly increased by exercise and by use of the brain itself in complex activities of work and fun.
   7. It is also well accepted that long periods of inactivity are not good for your health or brain functioning.

C. For people who have gotten into a condition where they cannot exercise very much, it may be that hyperbaric treatments may get them back to where they can exercise and get better. Also when the cost of time away from work or the

Only through Jesus Christ and many others was this Miracle possible!

8

costs of hospital types of treatment are considered, it may well be that it is in fact less expensive to go hyperbaric in the beginning. As the old saying goes, I think we, in many cases, are being penny wise and pound foolish in some of recent medical practices.

1. Hyperbaric oxygen therapy (HBOT) is a medical treatment that delivers 100% oxygen to a person within a pressurized chamber.
2. Each hyperbaric oxygen treatment is called a "dive." During treatment, 100% oxygen fills the hyperbaric chamber while atmospheric pressure is simultaneously increased. This therapeutic combination causes oxygen concentration within the body to increase 15 to 20 times normal. Increased oxygen concentrations help the body initiate cellular processes that can accelerate healing and aid in the recovery from certain conditions and illnesses.
3. HBOT is non-invasive, safe, and has few side effects.

BENEFITS of HYPERBARIC OXYGEN THERAPY

- Accelerates cellular renewal
- Supports growth of new blood vessels
- Promotes growth of new tissue
- Decreases swelling and inflammation
- Increases the body's ability to fight infections
- Helps to metabolize some toxin
- Potentiates antibiotic capabilities
- Stimulates collagen production

Hyperbaric oxygen therapy has been demonstrated to dramatically increase immune capabilities, assisting patients with problems ranging from chronic wounds to complex disabilities and neurological impairment. While HBOT has been used extensively by the international medical community for many years, its use is in its infancy stages, but rapidly increasing in demand, throughout the United States.

The basic principle behind hyperbaric oxygen therapy is easy to understand – oxygen is vital to the healing process. In normal conditions, only red blood cells have the ability to carry oxygen to injured parts. During HBOT, oxygen is dissolved in all body fluids – such as plasma, lymph, interstitial, synovial and cerebrospinal fluid. Increased oxygen levels, in turn, raise the body's ability to create new blood vessels, build new connective tissue, and foster the growth of new cells.

Rehabilitation time from injury has been accepted to have an intrinsically set rate. In other words – the body only heals at one speed. Although comfort measures and traditional therapies can be applied, the patient must basically wait out the predetermined healing time that nature has set for us. However, with the addition of hyperbaric oxygen therapy (HBOT), the previous standard of unalterable healing time has been revolutionized.

A new era in therapeutic treatment lies ahead as scientific data continually documents emerging uses and proven effectiveness of HBOT. Hyperbaric Therapy of the Low country utilizes state-of-the-art, fully computerized, cutting edge hyperbaric technology and adheres to industry safety standards.

///

SUMMARY OF RESULTS SO FAR

This first book is a brief account of me getting rid of Parkinson's disease and free of the Mirapex medicine that I quit taking gradually and that was used to combat my Parkinson's disease. In addition, I am still temporarily taking Azilect for the Parkinson's disease. The Azilect causes no problems.

1. My next door neighbor, Doctor Vern Gilbert a retired Internal Medicine Doctor has declared that I am free of Parkinson's disease.

2. My goal now is to get rid of any suggestions that the Parkinson's disease is not completely gone. Most of my current problems that make some say I am not rid of the Parkinson's Disease completely comes from not being as physically as fit as I can be. If it gets no better, I am functional and able to take on any mental job of my training.

   a. My physical ability is improving. I am now in a well- coordinated physical fitness program.

   b. I have a full scale treadmill in my home Super Google Style Office and physical training is no problem. Our cheery work environment keeps everyone at our home/business office engaged at least 90%. My internet search gave a 13% worldwide full engagement rate. We have fun and spiritual time.

3. Mental Functional Ability

   a. I am once again able to use the total Microsoft Office 2007 very well. I also am able to use Quickbooks Premier Plus Edition 2015 doing time, payroll, billing, and all other functions without any help from the Intuit Support Team.

    b. I am once again inventive and can put together proposals quickly and logically in many different areas.

4. IN THE FALL OF 2012 I WAS EFFECTIVELY DEAD AND AT PAIN LEVEL 10 AND ALMOST UNFUNCTIONAL MENTALLY. THE TREND WAS ALSO DOWNWARD RAPIDLY TO SURE DEATH AS MY DEAR MOTHER HAD EXPERIENCED. I SWORE TO MAKE THAT NOT POSSIBLE FOR OTHERS.

5. Looking Forward - I have put forth the new theory and way of treating almost all of these nerve diseases.

6. I have put forth the Theory that almost all the Parkinson's, Alzheimer's, fibromyalgia, and other such nerve damaging diseases are caused by insufficient blood flow to the nerves involved.

7. That we should fix the nerve damage and not treat with the medicines now used that do not fix anything and cause damages all their own that lead in most cases to downward movement in health and wellness and eventually to death.

8. That this nerve damage should be treated by increasing blood flow to the these nerves and also to the whole body through aerobic exercise whose benefits are:

    a. An in-shape body that also has a much sharper mind.

    b. An in-shape body that can work and play once more instead of heading sharply to bed confinement and death.

9. This simple treatment will cut medicine costs, medicine damage, and overall medical costs

10. This exercise treatment also will keep almost all diabetics free of neuropathy.

11. The net savings of adopting these programs will save 100's of billions of dollars.

THINGS THAT HAVE CHANGED AND THEIR ESTIMATED CHANGE AND DAILY VARIATIONS

ITEM	BEFORE PARKINSON'S	WITH PARKINSON'S + MIRAPEX + AZILECT	WITHOUT MIRAPEX[6]/ + EXERCISE[7] + AZILECT
COMPUTER ABILITY	100%	5%	100%
DAILY VARIATION	0%	0 TO - 100%	0 TO -20%
PERIODICITY		3 hrs	6 hrs[8]
EYESIGHT	Great[9]	NEEDED MAGNIFICATION	BACK TO NORMAL[10]

---

[6] Mirapex stopped gradually starting in September 2012, from 1.5 mg/day to 0 in November 2012. Mirapex had been started September 2006 at 1.0 mg/day. Azilect started on September 2008 at 1.0 mg/day and has not yet been changed. My removing Mirapex was supported by one person related to a friend, whose huge problems with Mirapex resulted in divorce and other bad things. The other support in getting rid of Mirapex came from my endocrinologist, Doctor Elaine K. Bunick, who said she knew of people who had bad reactions to Mirapex. In my doctor's visits, she had seen these features in me.

[7] **A referenced method of mice getting free of Parkinson's with aerobic exercise was used by me in about 2008 to essentially eliminate my bad shaking with my Mirapex. I include this reference to aerobic and other exercises effects on cognitive functioning to stimulate those interested to read all of the literature.** The clinical studies showed that various types of exercise, including aerobic, resistance and dance can improve cognitive function, although the optimal type, amount, mechanisms, and duration of exercise must be determined by a health team, who is supportive of this type of treatment. My theory has always been to do as much as you can and have fun when at all possible. Once fully tested, most will not quit because they feel so much better. I started long distance jogging and had to quit at 5 miles due to my knees, but once over the initial hurdle it was always very enjoyable.

[8] Due to pain pill coverage lapse every 6 hrs and is still happening.

[9] **Since Parkinson's inception, I have voluntarily stopped driving due to deterioration of space coordination of sights.**

[10] Lost most useful vision out of my right eye due to "Normal Optical Practices" that violated the manufacturer's recommendations which are as follows from the internet site (http://www.medsafe.govt.nz/profs/datasheet/p/Predforteophthsoln.pdf) on 4-14-2014,

ITEM	BEFORE PARKINSON'S	WITH PARKINSON'S + MIRAPEX + AZILECT	WITHOUT MIRAPEX[6]/ + EXERCISE[7] + AZILECT
		UP TO 200% With large fonts	
DRIVING	GREAT	UNSAFE & I STOPPED	READY TO RESUME
PAIN LEVELS			
Hyper sexuality[11]	0	5 to 10[12][13][14]	2 to 5[16][17][18]
General Body	0	5 to 10[15]	2[19]

"PRED FORTE® prednisolone acetate Datasheet Version 1.0" FROM THE MANUFACTURERS DATA, "Eye drops containing corticosteroids should not be used for more than 10 days except under strict ophthalmic supervision. If this product is used for 10 days or longer, intraocular pressure should be routinely monitored even though it may be difficult in children and uncooperative patients. Steroids should be used with caution in the presence of glaucoma. Intraocular pressure should be checked frequently.

[11] **"Loosening addiction's deadly grip", from "science & society," analysis. MBO reports VOL 7 | NO 2 | 2006; ©2006 EUROPEAN MOLECULAR BIOLOGY ORGANIZATION; pages 140 – 142. Recent research paints a picture of addiction as a progressive, chronic neurological disease that wreaks havoc with brain chemistry. In the second paragraph hyper sexuality is mentioned as one of the serious side effects. It has caused divorce, and other hugely serious problems. Consult the published literature for further information on the hyper sexuality side effect and many other very serious effects.**

[12] When lying in bed the hyper sexuality (primarily penile shaft) pain was the lowest. When standing up it was the worst and unbearable. The pain medications lowered this pain, but did not eliminate the pain to durable levels. Also the pain medicine is not at a constant level in the body and that affects the pain level strongly.

[13] **Professional journal articles citing hyper sexuality are included in the bibliography.**

[14] California class action lawsuits are cited in the bibliography.

[15] **The pain level was so severe that the first time on September 19, 2012 my wife took me to the Oak Ridge Methodist Hospital Emergency Room and the second time on November 10, 2012 the Emergency Squad had to haul me from my upstairs bedroom on a stretcher. Both times I was in such pain that I thought I was going to die. The ER write up was complicated by some other issues that were happening including constipation. The central problem was the Mirapex however.**

[16] University of TN Hospital/Doctor complex urologist Doctor Kim said my method of massage to get blood circulation greatly improved and thus supply oxygen to nerves was a good idea to try. No one else had approved or suggested anything else.

PROBLEM AND SOLUTION SUMMARY
TO PERMIT EARLIEST PUBLICATION

A. My assertion is that Parkinson's Disease has been removed from me and that I am now functioning again mentally and my strength, flexibility, and agility are improving. The full extent to which I may improve is yet to be determined. I estimate a full strength and flexibility recovery.

B. My mind is now working once again, and I can do most anything requiring my mind and have proven that assertion.

C. I believe that the Mirapex problem of hyper sexuality has been solved partly by body aerobic exercise and massage therapy of the area at home. This increases the blood supply to the damaged nerves and after some time heals the nerves.

D. The general previous solution methodology of using more pain pills has been logically destroyed.

E. In recent years physical therapy treatment has been reduced and pain pills have been substituted producing very bad results. These results are also very much more expensive in the longer run, because they effectively destroy the person using them.

F. Pain pills definitely have a place in medicine and in some cases may be the only solution for short term. In some cases this may also be true for long term therapy.

G. This country must get people off of their duff and moving much more aerobically, in strength training, and in flexibility.

H. All my assertions stated here are contained in the leading health care center publications, such as Johns Hopkins, Mayo Clinic, and the Cleveland Clinic.

---

[17] **Parkinson's Disease Society letter from a Mirapex damaged person, a nurse who is wife of a doctor, who did not think of any way to get help or to solve the Mirapex problem.**
[18] The Dagenhart massage therapy solution to the hyper sexuality problem is working and progressing to a complete solution, which will be published when more data is available. Estimated time to complete testing is 3 to 6 months, as extrapolated from other similar problems. The principle problem is how long it takes for the nerves to heal.
[19] **It took over 2 years to reduce the general worst body pain (no head pain ever noticed) to negligible levels today. The solution involved removing Mirapex medicine from being used and the application of aerobic exercise.**

Only through Jesus Christ and many others was this Miracle possible!

BAR CHARTS OF THE VARIOUS PAINS & THINKING ABILITY BEFORE PARKINSON'S, PARKINSON'S AT ITS WORST, AND NOW

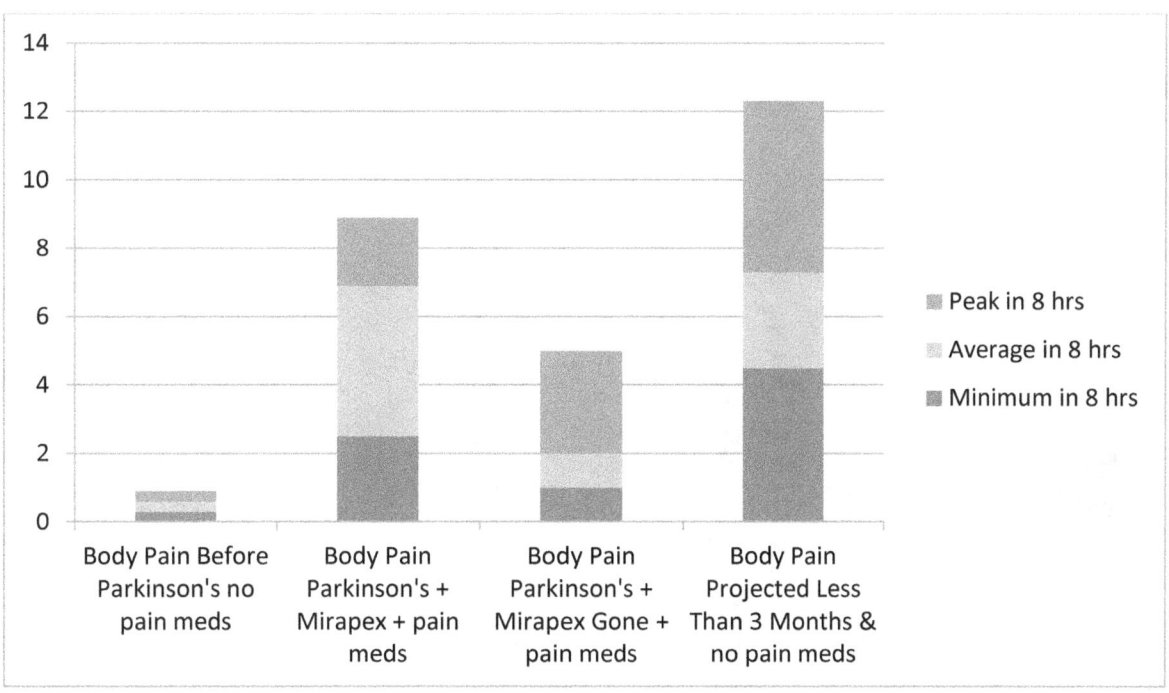

Notes:

1. Body pain during exercise and all other activities was normal before Parkinson's medicine Mirapex.

2. During the worst times with Parkinson's and medicine use of Mirapex the pain could go to 10 and be unbearable. Without the pain medicine of Hydrocodone at the level of 5 mg plus 325 mg acetaminophen every 6 hours or 4 times per day, I would not been able to survive and would not have wanted to survive. I would estimate that there were 4 hours of the 6 that were good and productive and 2 hours that were not very good. For me one more pill per day was definitely needed.

3. After stopping Mirapex gradually, the almost only pain left was the bladder and penis shaft areas. At the current time the only significant pain left is the penal shaft, which in the literature is called hypersexuality. I simply cannot think of a better description. The only thing missing is the mental loss of control during real sexual activity for some.

4. Physical and as vigorous an activity as I could stand was also helpful to me personally. As physical activity increased my mental ability greatly increased and my general body pain decreased to almost nothing.

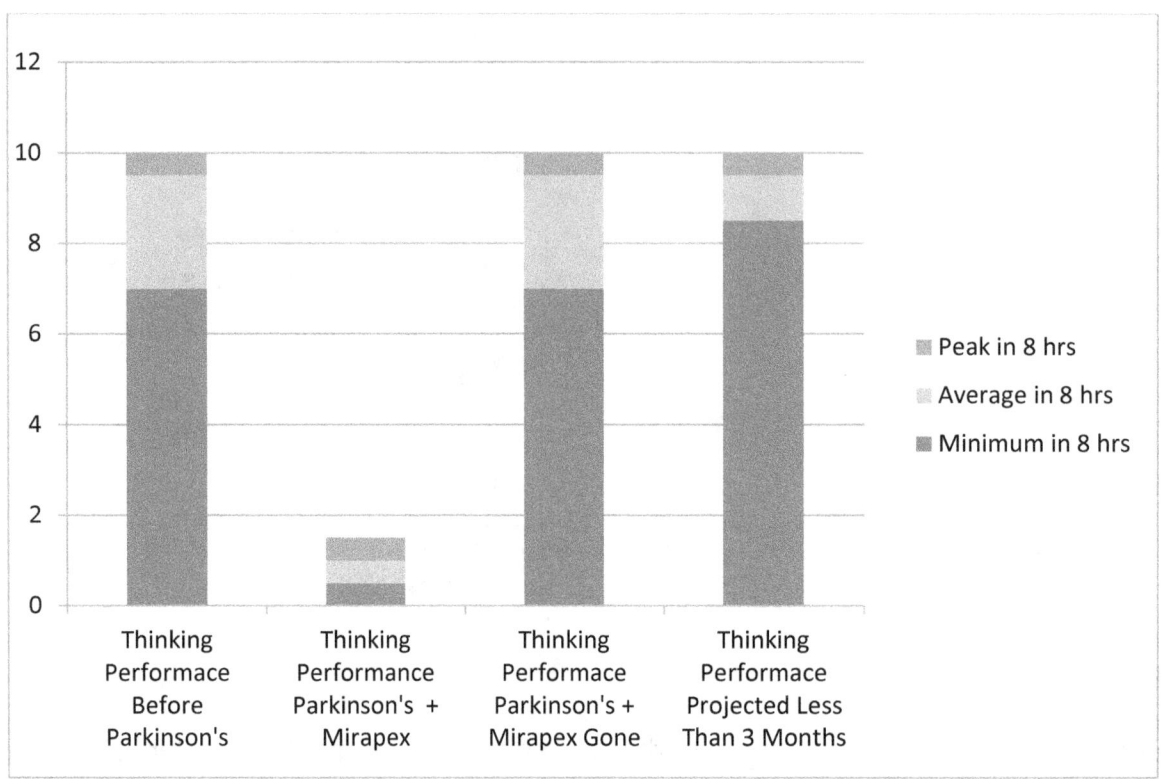

Notes:

1. I was innovative before Parkinson's and before using the medicine, Mirapex. My main holdback was not having venture capital or being permitted to spend much of anytime on any but prescribed program activities at The Oak Ridge National Laboratory.

2. To prove my former inventiveness, I have several documents that have been professionally published. I have a ¾ inch professional video of my invention of a car exactly like the present Toyota Hybrid. Mine was to be propelled by drive at each wheel and power would come from either a battery or preferably a rotating energy storage device. I have published information on such a device at a conference in Oak Ridge held by the Oak Ridge National Laboratory. Discussions within The Engineering Technology Division of ORNL confirmed that the opinion was that the breakup of such devices could be held to very low rates of

happening and confined within sensible housings by programmed breakup of the rotating device.

3. My renewed inventiveness is contained in ways to;

    i. Prevent the development of large forest and grass fires within very economically sensible means. Provisional Patent Granted.

    ii. A way to lower all kinds of operational disasters such as driver caused car crashes from alcohol, drugs, and fatigue. This prevention method also extends to all types of operational errors in trucks, airplanes, and ships for example. In process.

    iii. "There is more folks."

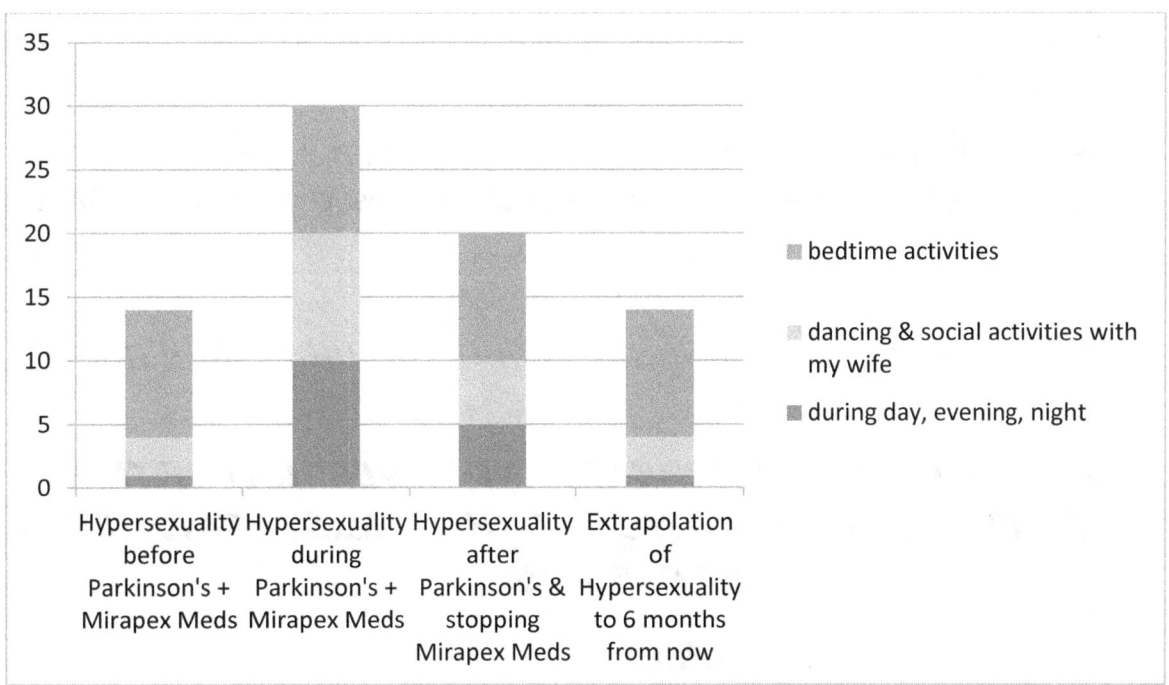

Notes:

1. This problem has been proven in successful court cases in the state of California to be caused by Mirapex.

2. My theory was agreed with during a Knoxville Pain Clinic Nurse Practitioner interview for pain medicines. She agreed that my assertion that the nerve damage by Mirapex could be interpreted by the brain as hypersexuality.

3. A Knoxville Urologist agreed that my proposed method of increasing blood supply by massage of bladder area and penis could provide the oxygen needed for nerve repair.

4. I have just been made aware of the detailed improvements in oxygen supply that can be proved by Hyperbaric Therapy. My one main question is - are there any bad side effects from using 100% oxygen atmosphere. If there are any, then I think the oxygen percentage could be lowered to a level where it was safe. Side effects from these rich oxygen atmospheres during treatment remain to be documented and other data taken at lower levels.

5. I see no reason why this data cannot be gathered in well controlled experiments with consenting patients and by guidance from one of the National Physicians Groups or maybe several of them.

6. The cheapest and most effective treatments perhaps could be had through wider use of Hyperbaric Therapy.

7. I do not dispute that some medicines are necessary, but that the Old Adage of "Keep It Simple Stupid, that I have always used and most certainly did at ORNL applies here also.

//

OUTLINE OF A COMING MORE EXPANDED VERSION OF THIS PARKINSON'S DISEASE SOLUTION WITH CONCISE STATEMENTS OF RESULTS

Chapter 1

Parkinson's diagnosis and history

- Was solidly diagnosed & treated in my loving mother by the National Institutes of Health & others.
- My mother died at The Oak Ridge Methodist Hospital in a horrible scene of Parkinson's disease and medicine side effects. I am devoted to making diseases like this essentially vanish and am now convinced that this is possible.
- A neurologist and all my other doctors have agreed with the diagnosis of Parkinson's disease in me for well over 8 years.

Only through Jesus Christ and many others was this Miracle possible!

//

Chapter 2

My Medical History in Brief

- Born on April 8, 1937. Home birth doctor attended in Stony Point, North Carolina.
- Polio in 1946 – no enduring symptoms, maybe because the hospital couldn't keep me still and in the bed. This was actively stated by the hospital doctors at that time.
- Diagnosed in June 1950 with Type 1 Juvenile Diabetes with a blood sugar of ~ 600. My HbA1c (3 month average of glucose) has always been 5.8 to 7.3 (1 exception was 8.3).
- Serious constipation problems since 1960 – solved completely October 2013 by using a variation of the advice from my daughter of stomach massage that I converted to something more fun -- The Dance WIGGLE. It replaced recently prescribed pills that were causing blood in my colon.
- Serious heart attack April 1993. A plugged upper left anterior descending artery. Rooted out by Doctor Jim Michel before stents and with the addition of cholesterol reducing medicine – no trouble since. About 1 month ago an incident at my Rotary meeting caused me to be transported to the Emergency Room and then a possible stent procedure. It turns out nothing was necessary in the heart. It was caused by something I ate is my conclusion. The hospital had no cause listed.
- Parkinson's disease -- neurologist diagnosed 2006
- Worst time in fall of 2012 and with reaction to Mirapex medicine
- Now mostly recovered.

//

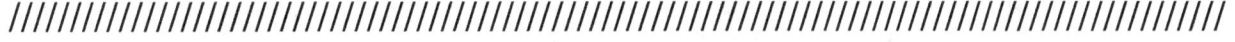

Chapter 3

Life Long Medical and Health Goals

- Since very early childhood was convinced from the Holy Christian Scriptures that Your Body is The Temple of God.
- Lifelong commitment to physical exercise, strength, aerobic, and flexibility
- Quit smoking at grade 3 after 3 packs of smoking with my buddies. I was convinced by a car going by as I walked to get another pack of cigarettes that the black smoke coming from the cigarettes could not be good for a person's body. At that time most people smoked and 86% of nurses and doctors smoked. My parents did also.
- After diagnosis of diabetes in 1960 – keeping my blood sugars as close to normal as possible was always my goal. While talking to a Johns Hopkins great doctor about my diabetes, he told me I was obsessive about my blood sugars. Being concerned is what has kept me alive.

//

Chapter 4

A Glimpse of Lifetime Results 1

- I have road driven and operated large farm tractors, backhoes, cars, large trucks, and taxies with only one very minor accident in my lifetime – At Radford College in Virginia on a rain slickened road, I slide into a car and damaged a rear taillight plastic lens. My attention had been diverted after leaving Sally off at Radford by three other pretty Radford College girls walking!
- I have repaired and operated systems from television high voltages in grade school to 150,000 volts at The Oak Ridge National Laboratory Fusion Energy Division safely
- In ~ 1968, I ran a 4 min 30 second mile against a Marine co-worker, who was maybe 1 second at most behind me.
- I have all my fingers, toes, etc. – nothing missing or non-functional. I am now planning to play the piano as my great Mother tried to make me be still long enough to learn – without any luck. My loving daughter has promised to try!
- I have no neuropathy, diabetic eye retinopathy, and have good feeling everywhere on and in my body.

- For example, I have successfully recently told a UT Hospital doctor that I had missed a half heart beat. He concurred by using an instrument output reading.

//

Chapter 5

The Worst Pain Level and Lowest Functioning Time

A Glimpse of Results – Fall 2012

- Was flat on my back at pain level 10 on the 0 to 10 Pain Scale at the Oak Ridge Hospital twice. Was at a 5-10 pain level most of the time even with pain medication.
- Was mostly wheelchair bound.
- It was extremely difficult to do much of anything on the computer in Microsoft Office or Quickbooks. Was able to do only absolutely necessary things with assistance.

//

Chapter 6

Getting Rid of Parkinson's

Fall 2013 – Preliminary Results

- On November 12, 2013 at Oak Ridge First United Methodist Church, I danced the rumba and waltz for 10 minutes unsupported with a female retired professional dance instructor (she and her husband, Baptists from Knoxville, teach dance at Oak Ridge First United Methodist Church every Tuesday from 6-8 pm in the Multipurpose Room – no charge).

Chapter 7

Results and Follow-on Programs 1

- My ability to operate Quickbooks, Microsoft Office, and such programs are now normal and quite competitive. I use all the features of all these computer programs now.

- I am embarking on a complete physical fitness program in Oak Ridge

- I have applied to, "Dancing with the Stars," on November 22, 2013 for the next season. I am sure this took them by surprise and will require some thinking on their part. Actually, I now see a marked shift in the participants to handicapped and older people on this, one of my favorite shows. I think I should get a fee or get to dance one season!

- Can you imagine the audience draw of someone who has gotten rid of Parkinson's, who will be competitive, but surely not win. The audience draw will be worldwide and a huge increase over normal.

- I have recently found out that my Oak Ridge National Laboratory retiree health insurance from The American Association of Retired Persons-United Healthcare pays for me and the whole family completely 24/7 at a local physical fitness facility in Oak Ridge. What a smart way for the insurance companies to save money in health costs.

- I am working now in several major areas.

- I am planning to spread my health results worldwide so that others can benefit.

- This first edition is short so as to get results out as soon as possible.

- A second edition will follow with expanded experimental data and results.

- A third edition is planned using data from a submitted request to several service clubs for a set of expanded tests involving Parkinson's disease with 100 participants, then tests of these methods on those with Alzheimer's, dementias of all types, fibromyalgia, and some others.

- In working as Chief Financial Officer with my daughter Pam's DayBreak Personal Services, I have gained insight into how to improve healthcare delivery. We are working with legislatures and medical staff to make more sensible things possible and so all work better as a team members.

- Almost all these suggested improvements will make people's lives much better, save vast amounts of money over their implementation costs, and will make medicine much more fun and enjoyable. These changes will achieve what the United States Obama Health Plan seeks – Health Care for All, while simultaneously achieving what the other political parties want – saving money and achieving a balanced budget. IT IS POSSIBLE AND I CAN GO TO THE BLACKBOARD AND IN A FEW HOURS SHOW HOW.

- An exciting possibility is that "The Rotary Club of Oak Ridge" is considering expanding my methods to a much larger of group of say 100 to test quickly and prove the applicability of these HEALTH METHODS in vastly improving the health of The United States citizens and then the World. Rotary is a worldwide organization of 1.3 million members of all faiths and none. We can test my results in 6 months from now and then have conclusive results in 12 months. We can then go worldwide.

- I believe this movement to much more exercise will greatly improve the health of the citizens of the United States and the world. Things like Parkinson's, Alzheimer's, dementia, fibromyalgia, type 1 & 2 diabetes diseases, and damages from them, will be greatly reduced. The wellness curve of the nation will be extended by 30 years instead of starting to shorten further as is happening now or worse live longer, but as sicker persons.

- Exercise combined with better diets, which our family has always followed will also produce huge wellness benefits. I saw a special on National Public Television, where they offer a video teaching these better diet methods for a donation of $60.

- The fall of 2013, I was among the 656 oldest living diabetics having diabetes the longest according to The Joslin Center. I don't know how that number has changed, since the start of 2016.

Chapter 8

Challenges to Christians and to the Whole Community

- You, like Reverend John Wesley, my Methodist Church's Founder, get on your horse and get out to the lost in spirit, health, and finances.

- IDEA 1 for SERVICE CLUBS AND CHURCHES – CHALLENGE THE ENTIRE COMMUNITY TO JOIN YOU. YOU WILL BE THE LEADERS AND DOERS in concert with them.

- This would complement the tremendous free clinic efforts of our Oak Ridge Community. We could maybe help with transport to the clinics. TRANSPORTATION IS A TERRIBLE PROBLEM FOR THE POOR. Make it free to those who cannot pay and/or accept work in payment such as helping with making their communities more beautiful and helping others.

- I have knowledge of demonstrated practical ways of involving many more – even some of those in retirement home settings for our efforts.

- The return on investment is solidly positive for all.

///

Chapter 9

Improving the Health Results for Diabetics, Parkinson's disease patients, and Everybody Diversified Consulting Inc. Medical /Business Division

- For ways that have been successful for me, I am publishing my results. For medical ideas, you will have to ask your medical team to okay, supervise, and take part in your actions. I have solid results that are backed up by Published Medical Journal articles and by such places as The Cleveland Clinic, Mayo Clinic, and The Johns Hopkins Hospital. I have an extensive collection of these articles, but certainly not all of them.

BRIEF BIOGRAPHY

William Kelly Dagenhart

1. Born in Stony Point, North Carolina on April 8, 1937. Lived there until just after Pearl Harbor December 7, 1941, when my father joined the war effort in taking one new Victory Ship down the Chesapeake Bay every day.
2. Was raised mostly in Maryland near Baltimore. Graduated from Riviera Beach Elementary, George Fox Junior High, and Glen Burnie High School in 1955.
3. Graduated in Physics with a minor in Mathematics from Virginia Polytechnic Institute in 1960. Married my wife Sally Rorrer Dagenhart on March 15, 1958 in Pulaski, Va. She went to Radford College where we met.
4. We had our first child Pamela in Radford on July 17, 1959.
5. We moved to Oak Ridge, TN on January 1, 1960 where I accepted employment at Oak Ridge National Laboratory for 37 years as a physicist.
6. I earned my MS in Physics in 1964 and my PhD in 1977 from the University of Tennessee in nuclear physics, while working full time. My theses were both done at the Oak Ridge National Laboratory.
7. My major projects at The Oak Ridge National Laboratory were:
   a. Thomas Wilson Whitehead and I designed a new magnetic configuration for the Calutron isotope separator, which was originally designed, fabricated, tested, and produced large amounts of U-235 for the first atomic bomb in 1945. With this new configuration we then designed its new associated source and receiver. We operated them in tests to prove their worthiness and 6 of the 255° New Isotope 40 ton Separators were installed.
   b. Whitehead and I then turned to designing a new 180° Oak Ridge Sector Isotope Separator. With the fabrication and installation complete it ran into significant beam instability problems during final testing. The focal point was moving erratically for about 4 ft during testing. This would have meant the complete dumping of this isotope separator if this problem had not been solved and nothing for an investment of approximately $10 Million in time and materials by ORNL. On a hunch, I solved a major beam instability problem in two days by using a guess in the hardware needed, super cooperation from the shop people, the R.E.D. mechanics, and the chemical operators, who installed the new equipment. No drawings were used with the first test, which succeeded royally; saving an estimated over $10-20 million program investment. With the new design, the separator produced isotope separator factor increases from approximately 200 for the original Calutron WWII design up to 500,000. I did my PhD Thesis on this Separator and on nuclear coulomb excitation cross section measurements made using the super high enriched targets that I made with this direct target deposition machine that used direct ion beam target

deposition. The cross section measurements were made using the Vandegraf High Voltage Accelerator at the main ORNL Campus.

c. In 1975 Research & Development money ran out from DOE in the ORNL Isotopes Division and I moved to the ORNL Fusion Energy Research Division. I was Project Leader for designing, installing, and operating the Medium Energy Test Facility, whose initial fast paced development and operation was to provide high power ion sources for a competitive shoot-off with Berkeley National Laboratory for the TFTR fusion research facility. The driving force was the goal set by DOE to have a fusion reactor in 15 years.

d. I then sold to the United States Army with a cold call that we could help with the Reagan Star Wars Program to shoot down incoming nuclear warhead fitted missiles. All of this work was also useful in fusion research.

e. As the Star Wars Program ended, I was almost immediately confronted with a request to lead a Nuclear Special Facility Clean Up situation that I estimated at a $50 Trillion risk level. The previous, well-qualified, company pulled out in a panic once they realized the risk involved and that there was no practical way to get coverage by any insurance company. I got to the site within about 6 hours after getting a 30 minute explanation of the problem and asked whether I would go. I said yes without any hesitation. I initiated and lead 15 major changes or program responses to this problem site in the 1½ years I was there.

f. I then moved on to The Enrichment Technology Division of ORNL. My first five years was to be an analyst of safety for the Uranium Gaseous Diffusion Plants in Portsmouth, Ohio and Paducah, Kentucky. The result was an enormous technical and practical safety education that compliments and extends greatly my dedication to safety on all fronts. The "What If" technical and practical input from on-site personnel in my opinion should be extended to input from all and to all industries. I have myself used this almost since I was born up until today. In a previous work situation, a craftsman responded to my question as to why he was doing it a certain way that I myself thought would not work. He responded that he had tried and made suggestions before and had been ignored. He said, "I just quit making suggestions then." I estimate that the neglected suggestion cost ORNL about $30,000 for that one item. There are only a few companies that listen and Toyota is one of them. They got more than a 9% return on investment by using this method.

g. My further developments in Engineering Technology Division involved a design just like the present Toyota Hybrid. I have myself a professional ¾ inch tape of this auto in simulated action, since the design was done for me on the outside. This system was dropped by the Department of Energy as being impractical. I just recently Googled that Switzerland had developed this same set of techniques into a practical bus propulsion system. They added an old time invention to the rotating gyro called a gimbal. The bus was competitive, but not cheaper to operate than gasoline or diesel fueled combustion engine powered vehicles. With the current ramping up of awareness of the dangers of the rising CO_2 in our atmosphere and its impending disaster, we should quickly get moving again on this effort. There are many companies offering this rotating energy storage concept.

h. I cold-called sold to the Portsmouth Gaseous Diffusion Plant Research Vice President, a possible improvement to the power system at Portsmouth. It involved a huge two billion centrifugal energy storage of electrical energy from cheap night time nuclear power and then converting it back into electrical power during the expensive daytime power period to supply power for the gaseous diffusion plant. After I, with a team of about 13 engineers, did a full feasibility study, I recommended that a slower development should occur to more accurately determine costs. At that time our team came to the conclusion that the payoff period was five years and the error bars on the payoff period too inaccurate to go forward that fast. The reason for dropping the project for Portsmouth was that the nuclear power locally dropped their prices. In doing so, that more than paid for our work. I have just Googled a device that employs all of the device attributes and design I proposed and is now commercially available for large power systems such as TVA in the Tennessee Valley Power System. All of these attributes were in my published conference paper.

i. I also have four scientific patents in the fusion technology arena. These were developed while at ORNL.

j. In the summer of 2014, I have begun applying for patents again and developing these patents into commercial devices. A United States Provisional Patent was filed in the summer of 2014 under my name, for stopping the initiation of big grass and forest fires. Several others are under development in completely different areas of engineering and science.

8. I have been retired since April 1, 1997.

9. After a bit of searching for employment again, I was selected by Battelle Memorial Institute to head a team that was seeking to win the contract for directing operation of the Y-12 Weapon's Plant in Oak Ridge, TN. This contract would have involved an operating budget, which was over $5 billion and a capital expansion/conversion budget of over $6 billion. I had always been doing work for ORNL, but located at the ORNL Facilities in the Y-12 Plant. I knew many of the people there and they are all top quality. I had even consulted a time or two with Dr. John Googan, a wonderful person. Just before making the contract competitive presentation to the Department of Energy in Oak Ridge, maybe only one day before, I developed what I have later had to name myself, DAGENHART'S EYE SYNDROME. My super, cornea eye specialist in Knoxville, Doctor David J. Harris, Jr., would not name it after himself. All other eye centers wanted to put grease on my eyes. His solution

was Prednisolone eye drops, which worked perfectly and restored my sight, which had almost been completely lost with eye watering continually, eye sensitivity forcing me to keep my eyes closed, and about 600/20 vision. Of course, they did not want a virtually blind man in this capacity, so we lost the job.

10. Pamela L. Dagenhart was born in Pulaski, VA on July 17, 1959. Son, W. David Dagenhart was born on May 14, 1962 when we lived at 140 Iroquois Road, Oak Ridge, TN. Keith Randal Dagenhart was born at the same location in February 22, 1964. Jonathan Kelly Dagenhart was born August 9, 1969. All were National Merit Scholars and went to college successfully.

11. Since getting out of graduate school, I have been involved in the Oak Ridge First United Methodist Church heavily. I am presently on the Social Concerns Committee of Oak Ridge First United Methodist Church.

12. I have been president of Remove Intoxicated Drivers of Oak Ridge/Anderson County since we lost our son, Keith Randal Dagenhart, to a car accident on August 9, 1982, when he was hit by a young girl head-on as she attempted to veer around 2 vehicles stopped in the road. Neither vehicle had anything to mark their presence, such as flashing lights, a white cloth, flares... He was wearing his seat belt and nothing was his fault. No alcohol was involved, but no other drugs were tested for at that time. I have been pushing for Drug Courts for our country, since about the summer of 2000 as a way of turning people around in their behavior instead of putting them in jail. I currently am working in consultation with Senator McNally, Head of The Senate Ways and Means Committee of TN. I have also recently been working directly with the Tennessee Governor's Offices.

13. I have been a Rotarian since about 1986 and am now in The Oak Ridge Rotary Club since about 2000.

14. Civic and business efforts I am involved in or are planning involvement in are;
    a. A patented idea for keeping forest fire initiating events from developing into large forest fires. I am currently in the beginning of negotiations with the California Governor's Office and others on these large tasks as a starting place.
    b. There are many other potentially patentable ideas that I now have and will once again be actively working and exploring their viability.

//

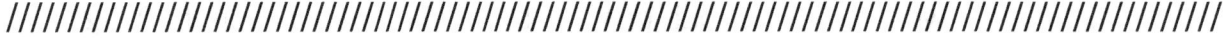

CHANGES IN HEALTHCARE I MAY HAVE GOTTEN STARTED OR HELPED ACCELERATE FORWARD and UPWARD

1. Last fall, Sally drove me to Boston's Joslin Diabetic Clinic, a 600-staff facility that does research and treatment for diabetics.

   I had been invited to take part in a long term study of why diabetics like me had lived longer than 50 years with little or no damages to our bodies. I was checked in and studied on Monday, October 14, 2013. So far my duration with Type 1 diabetes is 64+ years, with no damage that can be attributed to diabetes. At that time there were about 657 diabetics of longer duration. I have no neuropathy, no diabetic retinopathy; have all my appendages – fingers, toes, and such – in super working order.

   My lifelong habit was even in the beginning to hoe aerobically on our small farm. I have never given up that dedication, but keeping it up has been difficult lately due to health practices and practicalities of our budget and the medical practices of our nation.

   I suggested strongly that Joslin lead the way in adding exercises for all to their recommended health regime for diabetics and everybody. Exercise must be tailored to the health situation of the person.

   Joslin is now studying with a Ph.D. level team whether to add an exercise item to their formal long-term study.

2. This first book, my membership in Rotary and some terrific Rotary leadership may result in Rotary accepting my proposal to add exercise of all types to a Rotary backed long term study. For Polio, Rotary has had and still has the strong support from the Bill and Linda Gates Foundation at over the $300 million level. Rotary has also convinced many governments that it is in their strong interests to greatly raise funding for Polio eradication.

   There is growing support for health minded improvements in diet and exercise amongst others worldwide.

3. Locally, my daughter's DayBreak Personal Services has always had using the best methods in the health system as her goal.

Both Pam and I have personal experience in dealing with some of these terrible health problems and in seeking a better solution. Her problem is fibromyalgia and mine is diabetes and the residual problems from my bout with Parkinson's disease.

I have experienced huge improvements with these exercise methods and Pam is starting on an improvement path using exercise.

We had a client doomed to Hospice, who is now mentally up and functioning whole, as a person again. She went from essentially a "comatose type" situation to laughter now. There are many more cases like this.

Both ends of the spectrum...

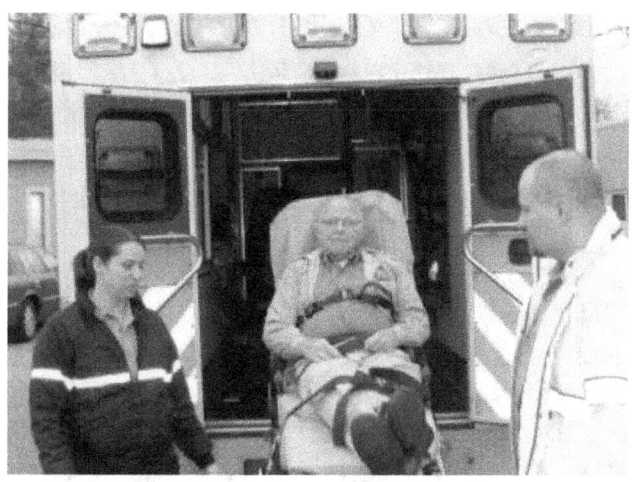

Transported by ambulance
pain level 10+
November 2012

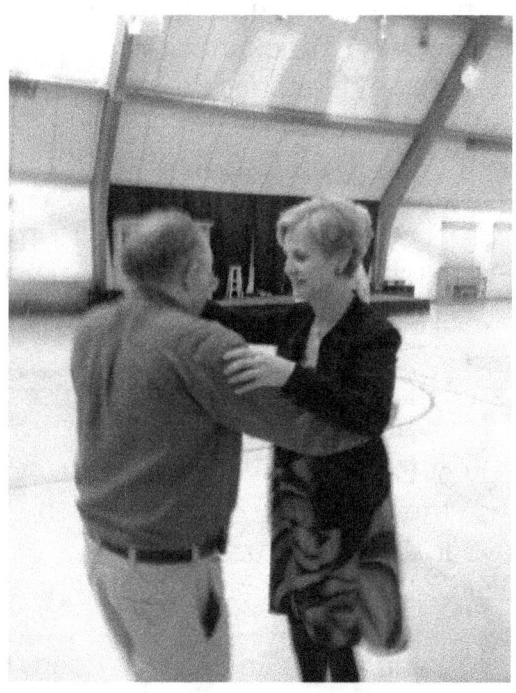

MIRAPEX GONE -- Dancing the waltz and rumba for 10 minutes at Oak Ridge First United Methodist Church on November 12, 2013 with Professional Dance Instructor. Photographed by Her Husband the Other Half of the Instructor Team.

Appendix A

A few Questions from Lynn Cardwell of American Reprographics Printing of Oak Ridge, Tennessee, a Rotarian reviewer and my answers

Kelly's Comments on
Lynn's Comments

1. What about a brief bio for the people that don't know anything about your background? Will do. Great comment.
2. Has anyone else tried your exercise regimen? How about getting some people from the local Parkinson's group to try it? It would give more credibility. I think to have more than one success story.
   a. After I pushed them, Vanderbilt has added exercise as one of their test variables.
   b. Cleveland Clinic and Mayo Clinic have aerobic exercise as a treatment, but not a solution yet on their website.
   c. There are United States Government backed demo projects. After I got by the first one in the list where they were using brisk exercises, I quit looking and put full time into my demo. My reasoning was backed by Doctor Kim, a urologist, whose office is at the University of Tennessee Hospital complex. My method states that the basic problem with many of these neurological problems is nerve damage due to lack of oxygen. I STATE THAT YOU MUST EXERCISE AEROBICALLY ALL OF YOUR LIFE FOR SOMEWHERE NEAR AT LEAST 1 HOUR DAILY. TO THIS MUST BE ADDED STRETCHING AND STRENGTH TRAINING. THE EXACT MIX HAS NOT BEEN DETERMINED. PIDDLING WILL NOT MAKE THESE GOOD RESULTS HAPPEN. I HAVE ADDED THESE REFERENCES. THESE EXERCISES GREATLY INCREASE THE BLOOD SUPPLY TO THE NERVES AND THUS THE OXYGEN SUPPLY NECESSARY FOR HEALING.
3. How about a brief description of your aerobic exercise and some logic about why it works? SEE #2
4. I don't see the analogy of Lazarus to your story. Maybe coming back from the dead? Maybe condense the Lazarus account down to 1 page and give the connection between your story and Lazarus.
   a. They thought Lazarus was dead and he would have been without Jesus' actions.
   b. I was at pain level 10 and in the Emergency Room two times within a month and could not have stood it much longer.
   c. Parkinson's itself is said to not kill you. However, Parkinson's with the same type of medicines did kill my Mother in the Oak Ridge Methodist Hospital.

They wanted to give more of the same medicines. You can extrapolate very well and come to your own conclusions.

d. I am now back to my former self. Maybe with even better inventive ability, working on the computer, and better in other aspects of life.

e. Physically I am not progressing anywhere as fast I could have or can at this time. I have self limited my driving in the past due to the medications diminishment of my visual coordination and other issues. I am now back and will be able to drive again eventually. THE MAIN PROBLEM HERE IS THAT I HAVE NOT BEEN ABLE TO GET TRANSPORTATION AND HELP IN MY PHYSICAL RECOVERY. THIS ISSUE IS ALSO REDUCED DUE TO MY REDUCED FINANCES, WHICH I THINK WILL SOON BE FIXED. I HAVE SPENT TIME DEALING WITH THESE FINANCIAL ISSUES. I HAVE MAYBE SIX POTENTIAL PATENTS FOR WHICH, I AM STILL LOOKING FOR HELP WITH VENTURE CAPITAL. I THINK THIS BOOK MAY SELL ENOUGH TO FIX THIS PROBLEM. I WILL BE ABLE TO GET ONE ITEM INTO PRODUCTION AND THEN WILL HAVE ALL THE FINANCING NEEDED TO DO THE OTHERS. BY PRACTICE IF NOT LAW, I WILL GO TO THE HEAD OF THE PATENT APPLICANTS LINE AND THESE ISSUES MAY BE SETTLED IN MONTHS NOT A YEAR OR SO.

f. MY FIRE PROVISIONAL PATENT HAS BEEN COMPLETELY FILED.

5. Is there any potential liability from Mirapex? I read some excellent reviews particularly from people with restless leg syndrome.

a. First there are huge Class Action Law Suits that have been won against Mirapex in California. I simply have not had time to look elsewhere for this type of litigation against the Mirapex medicine.

b. Of course to get approved, it must have serious side effects on less than 5% of users. I think just recently that there are those that claim rates up around 25% of users. I do not know where FDA action is on this issue.

c. When I go to such excellent health web sites as those of Cleveland Clinic and Mayo Clinics, they have aerobic exercise listed as one of the treatments.

d. I will make it clearer that I believe no one has ever claimed that aerobic exercise could clear up these health problems and then be stopped. THESE AEROBIC AND OTHER EXERCISES MUST BE DONE ALL OF ONE'S LIFE.

6. For a real controlled test of your theory, shouldn't you drop the Azilect? I'm shooting in the dark here, which is very risky. But is your recovery due to the exercise, the Azilect or both?

a. If I am unable to get rid of the Azilect, I will be perfectly okay and back to life once again.

b. Once I can get back to some resemblance of good physical shape and spending every minute struggling for economic survival. Pam's business has turned the corner and her net profit is up now by ~30% and will soon be where it should be.

c. I think that within 1 to 2 months, I will stop the Azilect too.

7. Doesn't Tennessee have some laws regarding the homeopathic practice of healing? Qualifications? Can anyone do it?

      a. From The Homeopathic Society Website -- Homeopathy is a system of medicine which involves treating the individual with highly diluted substances, given mainly in tablet form, with the aim of triggering the body's natural system of healing. Based on their specific symptoms, a homeopath will match the most appropriate medicine to each patient.

      b. AT FIRST I WAS DEAD SET AGAINST CALLING MY METHODS HOMOPATHIC – AFTER ABOUT A MINUTE OR TWO OF THOUGHT, I THINK YOU ARE DEAD RIGHT.

      c. As a runner, who hopes to be back soon, we have always claimed these health advantages. In about the third grade or so, I hoed on the small farm aerobically. I used simple logic going back to our beginning before civilization that people had to run aerobically to keep from getting eaten by the huge animals and to catch their food. Most did not do agriculture as I understand these peoples.

      d. The health clubs have always made these claims.

8. What about combining the support that I have, page 8, with page 9 Acknowledgements? There are a lot of the same people listed.

      a. Will do.

Thanks for your great suggestions. That was what I wanted from my reviewers.

Hopefully we will be able to get a much larger well controlled demonstration using the District Rotary Clubs. The assets will exist to do the demo at full speed and full requirements so that from there it will spread worldwide rapidly.

For anyone who would like to have input into this battle plan to improve our country and eventually the world's health, feel free to contact me.

Kelly Dagenhart
dagenhartwk@bellsouth.net
865-483-8801